# WHY DO
# PEOPLE
## CHOOSE TO SUFFER

## NORMAN LYONS SR. MSW

authorHOUSE®

*AuthorHouse*™
*1663 Liberty Drive*
*Bloomington, IN 47403*
*www.authorhouse.com*
*Phone: 1 (800) 839-8640*

*Published by AuthorHouse 05/19/2016*

*ISBN: 978-1-5246-0982-5 (sc)*
*ISBN: 978-1-5246-0981-8 (e)*

# CHAPTER I

I first would like to address, the person with an obsessive-compulsive disorder. According to the (DSM IV) diagnostic and Statistical manual of Mental Disorders. A person with this disorder is recurrent obsessions or compulsions (criterion A) that are severe enough to be time consuming (i.e., they take more than 1 hour a day) or cause marked distress or significant impairment. (criterion C). At some point during the course of this disorder, the person has recognized that the obsessions or compulsions are excessive or unreasonable (Criterion B). If another AXIS I disorder is present, the content of the obsessions or compulsions is not restricted to it(Criterion D).

The disturbance is not due to the direct physiological effects of a substance (e.g., a drug of abuse, a medication) or a general medical condition (Criterion E). Obsessions are persistent ideas, thoughts, impulses, or images that are experienced as intrusive and inappropriate and that cause marked anxiety or distress.

Compulsions are repetitive behaviors (e.g., hand washing, ordering, checking) or mental acts (e.g., praying, counting, repeating words silently) the goal of which is to prevent or reduce anxiety or distress, not to provide pleasure or gratification In most cases, the person feels driven to perform the compulsion to reduce the distress that accompanies an obsession or to prevent some dreaded event or situation.

After repeated failure to resist the obsessions or compulsions, the individual may give in to them, no longer experience a desire to resist them, and may incorporate the compulsions into his or her daily routines. This disorder will have significant intrusions, on a person's daily routines that, they frequently result in inefficient performance of cognitive tasks that require concentration, such as reading or computation. Such avoidance can become extensive and can severely restrict general functioning.

A recent analytic characterization that draws on elements of interpersonal conduct, self-esteem, and cognitive style has been presented by (Gabbard, 1994) in the following passage. Obsessive compulsive persons are also characterized by a quest for perfection. They seem to harbor a secret belief that if they can only reach a transcendent stage of flawlessness, they will finally receive the parental approval and esteem they missed as children. Most compulsive personality disorder individuals, seem to have a tendency to see things as all-or -nothing and in strictly black-and-white terms.

There is another concept, I feel has a major impact on anyone with this disorder, and that is, major control, and inconsiderate of others to follow very strict and harsh standards. These individuals are rigidly deferential to authority and rules. (Millon, 1969), put forth a theory-derived syndrome labeled "passive-ambivalence," a clinical pattern that paralleled in all major respects the character type variously called "anal," "compulsive." And "obsessional." To represent the deferential and self-constictin□□□□□□□□□□□□□□□□□□□□□□□□□□□□□□□□□□□□□□□□□ □□□□□□□□□□□□□□□□□□□□□□□□□□□□□□□□□□□□□□□□□□□ □□□□□□□□□□□□□□□□□□□□□□□□□□□□□□□□□□□□□□□□□□□ □□□□□□□□□□□□□□□□□□□□□□□□□□□□□□□□□□□□□□□□□□□ sume responsibility for most major areas of their lives. (Criterion 2). Adults with this disorder typically depend on a parent The four features we would abstract from the foregoing as characterizing the conforming (obsessive-compulsive) personality are: restrained affectivity (emotionally controlled: grim and cheerless), cognitive constriction (narrow-minded; overly methodical and pedantic in thinking), conscientious self-image (practical, prudent and moralistic), and interpersonal respectfulness (in-gratiating with superiors; formal and legalistic with subordinates).

# CHAPTER II

## "BORDERLINE PERSONALITY DISORDER"

I want to talk about these two disorders for a moment. Borderline Personality Disorder often co-occurs with Mood Disorders, and when criteria For both are met, both may be diagnosed. Because the cross-sectional Presentation of Borderline personality Disorder can be mimicked by an Episode of Mood Disorder. Just think for observation purposes, when we Meet people who display this kind of behavior, we need to be cognizant of the fact, these people are displaying symptoms which basically, they are not cognizant of. The person is just, being themselves actually.

What are you saying.? I am glad you asked. The person is revealing who they really are. Most borderlines are very needy people, and Will reveal their displeasure if you do not respond to their needs. We all Have needs, however, the Borderlines needs are eccentric. (e.g., deviating From an established or usual pattern or style of behavior, or, deviating from Conventional or accepted usage or conduct especially in odd or whimsical Ways.)

There is help for people with this disorder if they are willing to Seek help for themselves, noteworthy, most very seldom seek professional help unless, they happened to meet a healthy person who carefully suggest The idea, in a caring manner

If we really look at the context, in terms of, how these individuals really operate, in interpersonal relationships, we can better understand why most of these individuals have difficulty having a, meaningful, and healthy relationships with their partners. Interesting enough for the most part, these individuals very seldom feel that they need help, or need to seek professional help.

# CHAPTER III

## Alcohol-Related Disorders

In most cultures, alcohol is the most frequently used brain depressant and a cause of considerable morbidity and mortality. At some time in their lives, as many as 90% of adults in the United States have had some experience with alcohol, and a substantial number (60% of males and 30% of females) have had one or more alcohol-related adverse life events (e.g., driving after consuming too much alcohol, missing school or work due to a hangover).

Fortunately, most individuals learn from these experiences to moderate their drinking and do not develop Alcohol Dependence or Abuse. Some related Alcohol-Induced Disorders are as follows.

Alcohol Intoxication
Alcohol Withdrawal

Alcohol Intoxication Delirium
Alcohol Withdrawal Delirium
Alcohol-Induced Persisting Dementia
Alcohol-Induced Persisting Amnestic Disorder
Alcohol-Induced Psychotic Disorder, With Delusions
Alcohol-Induced Mood Disorder
Alcohol-Induced Anxiety Disorder
Alcohol-Induced Sexual Dysfunction
Alcohol-Induced Sleep Disorder

Because withdrawal from alcohol can be unpleasant and intense, individuals with Alcohol Dependence may continue to consume alcohol, despite adverse consequences, often to avoid or to relieve the symptoms of withdrawal. A substantial minority of individuals who have alcohol dependence never experience clinically relevant levels of alcohol withdrawal, and only about 55 of individuals with alcohol dependence ever experience severe complications of withdrawal (e.g., delirium, grand mal seizures). Once a pattern of compulsive use develops, individuals with dependence may devote substantial periods of time to obtaining and consuming alcoholic beverages.

Alcohol Abuse effects the individual school work, job performance either from the aftereffects of drinking or from actual intoxication on the job or at school; child care or household responsibilities may be neglected; and alcohol-related absences may occur from school or work.

The person may use alcohol in physically hazardous circumstances (e.g., driving an automobile or operating machinery while drunk). Legal difficulties may arise because of alcohol use (e.g., arrests for intoxicated behavior or for driving under the influence) Finally, individuals with alcohol abuse may continue to consume alcohol despite the knowledge that continued consumption poses significant social or interpersonal problems for them (e.g., violent arguments with spouse while intoxicated, child abuse).

When these problems are accompanied by evidence of tolerance, withdrawal, or compulsive behavior related to alcohol use, a diagnosis of Alcohol Dependence, rather than Alcohol Abuse, should be considered. Repeated intake of high doses of alcohol can affect nearly every organ system, especially the gastrointestinal tract, cardiovascular system, and the central and peripheral nervous systems. Gastrointestinal effects include gastritis, stomach or duodenal ulcers, and, in about 15% of those who use alcohol heavily, liver cirrhosis and pancreatitis.

## MAJOR DEPRESSION DISORDER:

Diagnostic Features:

The essential feature of Major Depressive Disorder is a clinical course that is characterized by one or more Major Depressive Episodes. Without a history of Manic, Mixed, or Hypomanic Episodes (Criteria A and C). Episodes of Substance-Induced Mood Disorder (due to the direct physiological effects of a drug of abuse, a medication, or toxin exposure) or of Mood Disorder Due to a General Medical Condition do not count toward a diagnosis of Major Depressive Disorder. In addition, the episodes must not be better accounted for by Schizoaffective

5

Disorder and are not superimposed on Schizophrenia, Schizophreniform Disorder, Delusional Disorder, or Psychotic Disorder Not Otherwise Specified (Criterion B).

Similarly, if manic or hypomanic symptoms occur as a direct effect of a general medical condition, the diagnosis of Major Depressive Disorder remains appropriate and an additional diagnosis of Mood Disorder Due to a General Medical Condition, With manic Features (or With Mixed Features) should be noted. (DSM IV, 1994). Associated features, Major Depressive Disorder is associated with high mortality. Up to 15% of individuals with severe Major Depressive Disorder die by suicide.

Epidemiological evidence also suggests that there is a fourfold increase in death rates in individuals with Major Depressive Disorder who are over age 55 years. Individuals with Major Depressive Disorder admitted to nursing homes may have a markedly increased likelihood of death in the first year. Among individuals seen in general medical settings, those with Major Depressive Disorder have more pain and physical illness and decreased physical, social, and role functioning.

Other mental disorders frequently co-occur with Major Depressive Disorder (e.g., Substance-Related Disorders, Panic Disorder, Obsessive-Compulsive Disorder, Anorexia Nervosa, Bulimia Nervosa, Borderline Personality Disorder). It is very apparent that, people with the above (Disorders), especially those who are substance abusers, other chemical abuse, such as, (marijuana, Cocaine, Amphetamine, Alcohol, and Heroin) Are subject to the diagnosis of, Major Depressive Disorder, Dysthymic Disorder, Schizophrenia, Delusional Disorder, and Psychotic Disorder not otherwise specified.

Much to my surprise, and maybe the reader of this book as well, anyone who abuses the above chemicals, is definitely a candidate for these disorders. I wasn't cognizant, of the fact that what I, at one time was putting in my system, was destroying some of my brain cells, which is very important for anyone to function on a meaningful level. The (CNS) <u>Central Nervous System,</u> and the Brain, is <u>how the human body, soul and mind operates.</u> Anything that interrupts the normal passages of messages to the CNS and then to the brain, will result in dysfunctioning, as oppose to normal functioning.

I had to get clean and sober first, finished my undergrad work, and then go on grad school and finished my Master of Social Work Degree, before I was exposed to this knowledge. Now, the readers of this book is aware (cognizant) of why I decided to share this pertinent information with others. Maybe, those who chance to read this book, will think twice, or three times, on continuing to use and abuse chemicals, if they really want to be a healthy individual.

I felt that, it was important for me to share this with you (the reader), because I care about people, mainly my black brothers and sisters, however, I care about people in general. I care so much, it motivates me to try and lead men and women to the Lord and Savior Jesus Christ. Had it not been for him (Jesus), when I cried out to God, and Jesus saved me, and turned my life around, and gave me a new beginning, a new look, a new walk, a new talk, and a new purpose in life with a new perspective, I would not be alive today, I know this without any doubt in my mind. I really am truly grateful to the Lord for what he has done for me, and what he can do for you, if you only believe.

Now, there are some people, who suffer from mental disorders without using drugs or other chemicals, these people need to take medication on a regular basis. When a doctor prescribe a medication for a patient, if the patient decides they do not want to take the medication, they will decompensate. (loss of physiological compensation or psychological balance) If you know that you should be taking medication, and you refuse to take it, you will loose your balance, in terms of, mental, or physical, you will definitely suffer, not the doctor, but you.

## BIPOLAR I Disorder

(Recurrent Major Depressive Episodes With Hypomanic Episodes)

Diagnostic Features: The essential feature of Bipolar II Disorder is a clinical course that is characterized by the occurrence of one or more Major Depressive Episodes (Criterion A) accompanied by at least one Hypomanic Episode (Criterion B) Hypomanic Episodes should not be confused with the several days of euthymia that may follow remission of a Major Depressive Episode. The presence of a Manic or Mixed Episode precludes the diagnosis of Bipolar II Disorder (Criterion C).

The symptoms must cause clinically significant distress or impairment in social, occupational, or other important areas of functioning (Criterion E) In some cases, the hypomanic Episodes themselves do not cause impairment. Instead, the impairment may result from the Major Depressive Episodes or from a chronic pattern of unpredictable mood episodes and fluctuating unreliable interpersonal or occupational functioning. Individuals with Bipolar II Disorder may not view the hypomanic Episodes as pathological, although others may be troubled by the individuals erratic behavior.

It is interesting to note, Individuals with the above disorders, at times will reveal their sickness unconsciously because for the most part, they will refuse to go and be treated. It is extremely difficult to connect with people with these kinds of problems. One day, they may be up, and the next day, they may be down and depressed, so it is difficult to know which person is going to show up the next day. It is not healthy for a healthy individual to become involved with people like this, in terms of, trying to establish a relationship, they are not mentally nor emotionally available to connect with you.

## "SCHIZOPHRENIA"

In individuals with a previous diagnosis of Autistic Disorder (or another Pervasive Developmental Disorder), the additional diagnosis of Schizophrenia is warranted only if prominent delusions or hallucinations are present for at least a month (Criterion F). The characteristic symptoms of Schizophrenia involve a range of cognitive and emotional dysfunctions that include perception, inferential thinking, language and communication, behavioral monitoring, affect, fluency and productivity of thought and speech, hedonic capacity, volition and drive, and attention.

The "psychotic dimension" includes delusions and hallucinations, whereas the "disorganization dimension" includes disorganized speech and behavior. Negative symptoms (Criterion A5) include restrictions in the range and intensity of emotional expression (affective flattening), in the fluency and productivity of thought and speech (alogia), and in the initiation of goal-directed behavior (avolition).

Delusions are another part of the Schizophrenic Disorder. For example, e.g., (a person who has this disorder may, believe that a stranger has removed his or her internal organs and has replaced them with someone else's organs without leaving any wounds or scars). This kind of delusion is considered to be a bizarre delusion.

It is very important to understand when a Schizophrenic began to hear voices, and began to experience auditory hallucinations. The voices are usually experienced whether familiar or not, they are perceived as distinct from the person's own thoughts. Threatening voices are very common.

Most Schizophrenic clients or patient's, involves dysfunction in one or more major areas of functioning (e.g., interpersonal relations, work or education, or self-care) (Criterion B). Functioning is clearly below that which had been achieved before the onset of symptoms. If the disturbance begins in childhood or adolescence, however, there may be a failure to achieve what would have been expected for the individual rather than a deterioration in functioning. Comparing the individual with unaffected siblings may be helpful in making this determination. Educational progress is frequently disrupted, and the individual may be unable to finish school. Many individuals are unable to hold a job for sustained periods of time and are employed at a lower level than their parents ("downward drift")

This next paragraph, may be interesting to those that wish to continue to use crack or amphetamine. Many different types of Substance-Related Disorders may produce symptoms similar to those of Schizophrenia, (e.g., sustained amphetamine or cocaine use may produce delusions or hallucinations; phencyclidine use may produce a mixture of positive and negative symptoms). The clinician must determine whether the psychotic symptoms have been initiated and maintained by the substance use. Ideally, the clinician should attempt to observe the individual during a sustained period (e.g., 4 weeks) of abstinence.

However, because such prolonged periods of abstinence are often difficult to achieve, the clinician may need to consider other evidence, such as whether the psychotic symptoms appear to be exacerbated by the substance and to diminish when it has been discontinued, the relative severity of psychotic symptoms in relation to the amount and duration of substance use, and knowledge of the characteristic symptoms produced by a particular substance (e.g., amphetamines typically produce delusions and stereotypies, but not affective blunting or prominent negative symptoms).

This tells me, and you, the reader of this important text that, by giving up the crack and other substances, the addict/alcoholic may have a chance to experience a decent and healthy life, not withstanding, giving their life to the Lord Jesus Christ for permanent deliverance from a life of damnation and shame. A life of demonic controlled by substances, You pick up the drug, and then the drug picks you up, and totally controls your life, if you choose to call this type of living a life. Most inmates, who are honest with themselves and others, including their counselors, will tell you when they got arrested, there was induced before the crime was committed. I was ministering one Sunday morning, and I asked the question to about 50 inmates who were present at the service, give me a show of hands of those who were using a substance, just before they were arrested. Not surprisingly, 90% of the inmates raise their hands. Again, so why do people choose to suffer?. Most Schizophrenic's are able to function, and even work, providing, they are willing to take their medication as prescribed by their Physician.

## "AVOIDANT PERSONALITY DISORDER"

According to (Millon, 1969), both sets of contradictory findings are correct. If viewed in terms of the distinction between active and passive detachment. Both detached patterns, passive (schizoid) and active (avoidant), are disposed toward the more severe schizophrenic disorders. One group, the passive or schizoid-will display chronic underreactivity, affectivity, deficit, cognitive slippage, and interpersonal indifference; whereas the other-the active, or avoidant-will show up as chronically overreactive and hyperalert, with affective disharmony, cognitive interference, and interpersonal distrust among their major features. (Millon, 1969)

The first portrayal that approximates the actively detached character of the avoidant was described in 1911 by Bleuler in his initial formulation of the schizophrenic concept. Discussing several of the contrasting routes that often lead to the psychotic syndrome, (Bleuler, 1950) recorded the early phase of certain patients as follows: There are also cases where the shutting off from the outside world is caused by contrary reasons. Particularly in the beginning of their illness, these patients quite consciously shun any contact with reality because their affects are so powerful that they must avoid everything which might arouse their emotions. The apathy toward the outer world is then a secondary one springing from a hypertrophied sensitivity.

Another early description that coincides in certain respects with the avoidant trait constellation was presented by (Schneider, 1923/1950) in his conception of the aesthenic personality. Although aesthenics are noted best by their extraordinary attention to and hypochrondriacal concern with bodily functions, this basic preoccupation extends into the psychic realm as well. Schneider described this feature as follows. Just as the aesthenic patient no longer takes his bodily functions for granted so he loses the normal, carefree attitude to psychic functions--. All this is due in the first place to the chronic habit of self-investigation. Psychic functioning as with bodily function becomes interfered with and starts to falter... feelings do not seem genuine, relationships appear lifeless and void... (Schneider, 1923/1950)

All human activity needs a certain psychic half light or chiaroscuro if it is to be experienced as an integral part of the self. Actions tend to disintegrate if full attention is focused on them in the same way as the body ceases to function smoothly if it is subjected to too much conscious interference. What Schneider is saying another way is, <u>if this kind of client begins to experience too much consciousness, they become frightened and will shut down altogether, because it is too much for this person to handle</u> comfortably.

We need to know this, in terms of, meeting new people in our quest for relationships, this is something that will not go away, if anything, it will get worse. The person will make the new partner uncomfortable, and they will begin to wonder, what is going on, did I do something to initiate this kind of response?. Descriptively, both (Reich, 1933) and (Menninger, 1930) addressed what we would now consider to be characteristics of the avoidant personality. Reich spoke of the following type:

This erects itself as a hard protective wall against the experiencing of infantile anxiety and thus maintains itself, notwithstanding the great forfeiture of joie de vivre which this entails. If a patient having such a character enters analytic treatment because of some symptom or other, this protective wall continues to serve... and it soon becomes apparent that nothing can be accomplished until the character armor, which conceals and consumes the infantile anxiety, has been destroyed. (Reich, 1933)

In a similar fashion, Menninger (1930) addressed a character type also akin to what we speak of today as the avoidant personality. He terms them "Isolated Personalities,". Among the personality types prone to failure in social adjustments... analysis discovers that these are really of two sorts. Some are "temperamentally" unsocial and really prefer to be left out of it... The other group is made up of wistful "out-siders" who long to dive into the swim and either don't know how or are held back by restraining fears which have been inculcated.

Lorna Benjamin (1993) did further work on the avoidant, and the following is some comments on the avoidant from this orientation, Benjamin writes: There is intense fear of humiliation and rejection. To avoid expected embarrassment, the AVD with-draws and carefully restrains himself or herself. He or she intensely wishes for love and acceptance, and will become very intimate with those few who pass highly stringent tests for safety. Occasionally, the AVD loses control and explodes with rageful in-dignation.

Expects to be degraded and humiliated by people, and so he or she refuses any assignments that might involve increased interpersonal contact and the associated likelihood of mockery, or the possibility that someone might say, "I don't want to deal with this (avoidant) person." Employing the factor analytic methodology to the study of personality disorders, Costa and Widiger (1993) have provided a latent mathematical model as a means of making explicit the underlying trait combinations from which the various disorders may be derived. In addressing the features that underlie the avoidant personality, Costa and Widi-ger point to the following trait combinations:

From the perspective of the FFM, AVD involves (a) introversion, particularly the facets of low gregariousness (no close friends, avoids significant interpersonal contact, and unwilling to get involved with others): low excitement seeking (exaggerates potential dangers, difficulties, or risks in doing anything outside of normal routine): low activity (avoidance of social and occupational activities, and canceling of social plans): and low assertiveness: and (b) neuroticism, particularly the facets of vulnerability, self-consciousness, and anxiety (e.g., easily hurt by criticism and disapproval).

Four criteria were proposed in Modern Psychopathology (Millon, 1969) The following are the four types:

1. Affective Disharmony (confused and conflicting emotions).
2. Cognitive interference (persistent intrusion of dis-tracting and disruptive thoughts).
3. Alienated self-image (feelings of social isolation: self-rejection).

4. Interpersonal Distrust (anticipation and fear of humiliation and betrayal).

According to the DSM IV, 1994), The avoidant Personality Disorder patients, have disharmony when it comes to (object relations), it is believed, most, if not all AVD patients did not have good relationships with their parents. Parents disregarded them in their growing and developmental stages of life, as a consequence, they learned how to cope or survive with this unusual high volume of stimulation. Thinking about this for a minute, made me pause for a question, in terms of, maybe the parents of the AVD, had parents which were not emotionally available for them, so in effect, he or she never received something, how can you give what you never received yourself. It would be extremely difficult to do.

For the most part, Avoidants see themselves as socially inept and inferior. Their self-evaluations judge them as personally unappealing and interpersonally inadequate, and they devalue whatever achievements they have attained. Most fundamentally, they find valid justifications for their being isolated, rejected, and empty.

Avoidants describe themselves typically as ill at ease, anxious, and sad. Feelings of loneliness and of being unwanted and isolated are often expressed, as are fear and distrust of others. People are seen as critical, betraying, and humiliating. With so trouble-laden an outlook, avoidants understandably show interpersonal aversivness in their social behavior.

Avoidants describe their emotional state as a constant and confusing undercurrent of tension, sadness, and anger. They feel anguish in every direction they turn, vacillating between unrequited desires for affection and pervasive fears of rebuff and embarrassment. Not infrequently, the confusion and dysphoria they experience leads to a general state of numbness.

As noted, avoidant personalities have a deep mistrust of others, and a markedly deflated image of their own self-worth. They have learned to believe through painful experiences that the world is unfriendly, cold, and humiliating, and that they possess few of the social skills and personal attributes by which they can hope to experience the pleasures and comforts of life. (DSM IV, 1994)

They anticipate being slighted or demeaned wherever they turn. They have learned to be watchful and on guard against the ridicule and contempt they expect from others. They must be exquisitely alert and sensitive to signs that portend censure and derision. And, perhaps most painful of all, looking inward offers them no solace because they find none of the attributes they admire in others.

Their outlook is therefore a negative one: to avoid pain, to need nothing, to depend on no one, and to deny desire. Moreover, they must turn away from themselves also, away from an awareness of their unlovability and unattractiveness, and from their inner conflicts and disharmony. Life, for them, is a negative experience, both from without and from within.

Oldham and Morris (1990) characterize the "vigilant" and the "sensitive" styles by the following: Nothing escapes the notice of the men and women who have a Vigilant personality style. These individuals possess an exceptional awareness of their environment. Their sensory antennae, continuously scanning the people and situations around them, alert them immediately to what is awry, out of place, dissonant, or dangerous, especially in their dealings with other people.

Sensitive people come into possession of their powers when their world is small and they know the people in it. These men and women- although they avoid a wide social network and shun celebrity-can achieve great recognition for their creativity. Nestled in an emotionally secure environment, with a few dear family members or friends, the Sensitive style's imagination and spirit of exploration know no bounds. With their minds, feelings, and fantasies, Sensitive people find freedom.

Another characterization of the avoidant style may be found in Millon et al. (1994), where the primary features are a "hesitating" pattern of social relatedness, an unsureness of one's acceptance, and a general feeling of unease and self-consciousness. Despite the features noted, these hesitating avoidant individuals may function competently in secure settings.

These persons have a tendency to be sensitive to social indifference or rejection, to feel unsure of themselves, and to be wary in new situations, especially those of a social or interpersonal character. Somewhat ill at ease and self-conscious, these individuals anticipate running into difficulties in interrelating and fear being embarrassed. They may feel tense when they have to deal with persons they do not know, expecting that others will not think well of them. Most prefer to work alone or in small groups where they know that people accept them. Once they feel accepted, they can open up, be friendly, be cooperative, and participate with others productively.

This next section will deal with some other types of Avoidants, adolescent's, adult subtypes, and the Conflicted Avoidant. In what he has called the "inadequacy syndrome," (Millon, 1969) describes the avoidant constellation as seen in adolescence. These youngsters are characterized by low self-esteem, an awkward self-consciousness, a timorous and hesitant manner in social situations, and a tendency to view themselves as incompetent, unattractive, clumsy or stupid. These youngsters feel that they cannot "make the grade," become a part of the peer in-group or be sought after and valued in the competitive give-and-take that characterizes adolescent relationships.

They dread facing the social responsibilities and expectations that society has established for their age group and are fearful that they will falter in finding a mate, getting a job and so on. In short, they lack the confidence that they can function and be accepted on their own. These youngsters do not question or reject the established values and goals of the larger society; they very much wish to achieve them and be considered "regular guys" or attractive girls. However, they experience repeated failures in their quest and slip into increasingly more isolated behaviors, preoccupying themselves with watching tv, day-dreams of glory and other forms of fantasy escape. (Millon, 1969).

The Adult Subtypes: Avoidant characteristics often acquire subsidiary features as they begin to withdraw socially and experience critical and unsupportive responses from others. (Millon, 1977, 1987, 1994) in Research shows that profiles including the avoidant pattern are shared most often with Schizoid, Dependent, Depressive, Negativistic, Schizotypal, and Paranoid Personalities.

When they begin to exhibit some of these associated personality features, the moods and actions that give a different coloration from the original traits that characterized the avoidant at the start. Insidiously developing features combine with the avoidant pattern and express themselves in a number of the subtypes discussed next.

Before we get into the next phase of the text, I want to address, and argue, in terms of, the difference in the population, and ethnic background of, not only these adolescent's, but also the adult subtypes. We need to look at the history and social background of the black adolescent and/or adult blacks. For the most part, blacks have been exposed to prejudice, racism, and 2nd rate education, for most of their earlier education years. This doesn't mean that, we as blacks cannot measure up to the task, however, the field of, or should I say, the education process for blacks in these United States have been for the most part, unequal from Pre-k to the 12th grade.

What I'm saying is, if the child (black) have not had the encouragement, motivation from the home, from the ground up, chances are, they will not be able to compete with their peers. Case in point, why bus a child from a good school area, into an area where he/ or she will not be exposed to higher educational processes, as the white or elite family child. In terms of funding for chartered schools, The funding is being taken from the regular public schools, and transferred into the private or chartered school areas. (think about that).

The better the private schools, the better, consequently the response from the student. Private schools have a much improved better educational process, in terms of, educating the student. The teacher's are better credentialed. Private and chartered schools, most always hire the best-credential teachers for their staff, that is the purpose for the extra funding, taken from the public school system, and transferred over to the private school.

In this process, in terms of education for the black child, the prognosis for this black child to be able to compete with his/her peers, is unlikely, mainly, because the earlier ground work was already laid for the child to not be able to compete with his or her peers, mainly because it was designed that way by the (dominant culture, white man). Wake up America, not much has changed since slavery, in these United States of America.

Now, in terms of fairness, if you really want to start out fair and balanced, let all children, regardless of race creed or color, and/or ethnic heritage or background, start equal in every phase of the educational process, and I guarantee you, the result will manifest itself in the grading process. In other words, if you start right in anything in life that one intends to accomplish a meaningful goal, chances are, you will enhance the child's efforts to success and self-esteem.

Most best credential teacher's, will demand the best pay for their work. The system has resolved to, take funds from the public school system and transfer these funds into the private school system, is this fair.? Of course not, however, if the legislature body in these United

States ignore this major problem, in terms of educating the black child, and any other minority population for that matter, the result will always remain the same, as designed by the dominant culture (white man.) We, the public, hear these talk shows about fair and balance, what is so fair and balance about this, I will tell you (nothing).

So you might say, what is the answer to all of this.? I am glad you asked. First of all, the black parent has to start out instilling into the black child, self-esteem. Let the child know, he or she is somebody and not nobody, like the dominant culture wants to project to society. In fairness, speaking of fair and balance, Our black children need less time watching tv, and more time devoted to homework from school. We need more parents (black) to be emotionally involved in their child's educational process. We need better monitoring tactics set up in the black home environment, in terms of, home work complete, now let me check and see how correct the home work is, and if so, give positive feedback to the child to empower him or her to continue the good work. Once the child see that his or her parent is concerned about their school progress, the child will inculcate the same process for his or her own motivating intent.

The work of (Bowlby, 1969, 1973, 1980) presented the notion that two fundamental personality variants experience the intensity of "loss" to an extent that produces a deep feeling of depression. Thus, Bowlby describes those who are "anxiously attached," at the one extreme versus those who are "compulsively self-reliant" at the other. According to Bowlby, excessive self-reliance is merely a defensive action against the experience of early loss and frustration, a response against the possibility of being drawn into dependency and care-taking roles for others.

By contrast, those who are "anxiously attached" seek interpersonal closeness at almost any cost, becoming increasingly dependent on these figures for their security, and resulting in a deeper concern about the stability about these relationships. This contrast of two depressively inclined character patterns is seen more clearly in the work of Beck (1983) and Blatt and Schichman (1983).

S. Blatt (1974) formulates his notions as follows: A character style in which there is unusual susceptibility to dysphoric feelings, a vulnerability to feelings of loss and disappointment, intense needs for contact and support, and a proclivity to assume blame and responsibility and to feel guilty. While types of depression are probably interrelated on a continuum, a simple or "anaclitic depression" describes an infantile type of object choice in which the mother is sought to soothe and provide comfort and care.

This type of depression results from early disruption of the basic relationship with the primary object and can be distinguished from an "introjective depressio," which results from a harsh, punitive, unrelentingly critical superego that creates intense feelings of inferiority, worthlessness, guilt, and a wish for atonement. (S. Blatt, 1974).

A. T. Beck & Freedman, (1976, 1983, 1990) Beck proposes that helplessness lie at the center of depressed personalities. In his theoretical model, Beck postulates the presence of underlying irrational schemas that derive from early developmental experiences. Two such schemas related to personality styles are detailed (beck, 1983).

The first he terms sociotropy, characterized by dysfunctional beliefs associated with the need for love and approval (e.g., I am worthless if everyone doesn't love me). The second personality schema is termed autonomy and is characterized by deep perfectionistic beliefs (e.g., If I make a mistake, I am a worthless person). Although Beck does not view these two cognitive schemas to be fixed personality types themselves, one may dominate an individual's cognitive functioning to a marked extent and ultimately produce exaggerated perceptions and emotional responses. Beck writes:

Sociality (sociotropy) refers to the person's investment inpositive interchange with other people. This cluster includes passive receptive wishes (acceptance, intimacy, understanding, support, guidance); "narcissistic wishes" (admiration, prestige, status); and feedback---validation of beliefs and behavior.

The individual is dependent on these social "inputs" for gratification, motivation, direction, and modification of ideas and behavior. The motif of this character is "receiving." Individuality (autonomy) refers to the person's investment in preserving and increasing his independence, mobility, and personal rights; freedom of choice, action and expression; protection of his domain; and defining his boundaries.

The person's sense of well-being depends on preserving his integrity and autonomy of his domain; directing his own activities; freedom from outside encroachment, restraint, constraint, or interference; and attaining meaningful goals. The motif of this cluster is "doing."

In contrast, the healthy individual will seek help for themselves. The other mode is, the mode of denial. Family and friends of this sort, may suggest to this type, maybe you need to talk to a professional and get some feedback, in terms of, why you continue the same behavior, knowing that you are miserable, and make family and friends, uncomfortable around you.

I think, the most difficult thing for a person of this type, is to, admit that something is wrong with me, or they are hard press to give in to defeat. This type of person is a prime ideal person of why I chose to write about. "Why People Choose To Suffer."

Most of these disorders, may be grounded at a very early stage of development, termed the sensory-attachment stage. It is at this time that children acquire experiences, through parental feeling and behavior, that their environment is receptive and caring or indifferent and distant. During this period, children learn to discriminate pleasurable experiences from painful ones. (Millon, 1996).

Fundamental feelings of security and attachment result from an adequate level of sensory gratification and nurturance. However, a failure to experience clear and unequivocal signs of warmth and acceptance at the sensory level may create fundamental feelings of insecurity, emotional detachment, and isolation.

If a child, who grows into adulthood, never received the proper love and caring, nurturance, security and attachment to object relations (parent), the child will evidently grow into a pattern of behavior, that will emulate his or her earlier developmental experiences. (e.g., imitate the same behavior which he or she is accustomed to.) The individual will become congruous, and conform to the situation as their usual pattern.

## "LOSS OF SELF"

Central to this period of development, is the emergence of a clear and cohesive sense of self, an inner representation of who the person is and who the person may wish to be. Such self-image representations may be either highly accurate or grossly distorted. What we find among depressive personalities is a judgement that one is valueless and worthless, inadequate and unsuccessful in all aspirations, a barren, sterile, impotent person who is both inconsequential and reproachable.

Primary, in this regard is the continuing feeling of not being loved, perhaps, more important, not ever being loveable. It is during and immediately post puberty and into early maturity that the mental image of "self" comes to be firmly embedded. As a consequence of earlier deprecations of self by others, followed by having fallen short during puberty, a sharp schism between self-image and "ego-ideal" becomes established; that is, the values and aspirations one desired for oneself are no longer possible to achieve. The split between reality and ideal is irremediable. (Millon, 1996)

It is the disparity between being and what might have been that the depressive believes has been severed forever. No cohesion can take place, no integration can occur between one's real self and one's ideal self. This everpresent cleavage in one's psychic makeup results in a sense of emptiness and loss, a loss not of others, not of parts of self, but of the very essence of self. Again, depressives feel helpless and hopeless about overcoming this schism. It remains an undercurrent that persists in creating gloomy moods and depressive cognitions.

Depressively prone youngsters not only allow themselves little pleasure, but are self-punitive and self-sadistic. Increasingly distressing though introspection may be, these children continue to find the reality of self to be despicable and condemable. Wherever they go, the despied self is inherent, an everpresent and condemned existence. Such introspection disrupts their cohesion and uncovers a fragile psychic state that produces a chronic series of depressogenic feelings, experiences, relationships.

Now, the confusion comes into play when, a person with this disorder meets a healthy person, who received love, nurturing experiences growing up as a child in his or her earlier environment, and also wants to be loved, and tries to give love and be intimate with this new person in their life but can't.

## "SELF DEFEATING BEHAVIORS"

One of the most obvious example of self defeating Behaviors is the jail and prison population. The recidivism Rate for this population is about 75% repeat offenders.

When you think about what this population have to go through, it makes you wonder how would anyone want to repeat this Negative, demeaning experience all over again. I have spoken to this group on many occasions, and it is disturbing when you hear some of the excuses an inmate will give you.

For the most part, many inmates just give up on attempting to change their behavior, or lifestyle. I, even had one inmate tell me that, I only feel comfortable when I am in prison. I do not have any skills, no higher education or degree, this is all I know. I would argue, This is all you want to know, most inmates have given up on hope, and refuse to even try and change their life for the better.

Life is full of choices, the result of any experience, is basically, the consequences based on the choice we made to the end result. The easiest thing for anyone to do is, give up on life and themselves. What helped me in this decision making process, I really got tired of being sick and tired of doing the same thing, and expecting a different result. The result is always the same when you refuse to change your behavior.

I recommend, let go and let God. God did for me, what I could not do for myself. I prayed to God for deliverance from the addiction of alcohol and marijuana abuse. I believed that God could and he did, remove this devastating disease from me, July 31, 1973. I have been blessed, not to have picked up the above since this date. I had been in the Ministry once before, and I experienced a state of backsliding from the will and faith in God. I then asked God, to forgive me for falling back into a world of sin and shame. God, for Jesus Christ, (His Son) sake, forgave me and restored me back in the fellowship with him.

I have been on fire for the Lord Jesus Christ ever since. God have put me in a prison Ministry, and I feel so blessed to have this opportunity to witness for the Lord, and to try and win souls for Christ. One of the major prophets Isaiah 55:6 said, "Seek ye the Lord while he may be found, call ye upon him while he is near." The prophet Jeremiah 29:13 said, "And ye shall seek me, and find me, when ye shall search for me with all your heart." Many have tried other avenues of or for relief, but have not been successful. I know from empirical knowledge this works, I was fortunate to lived the experience.

Anyone who is suffering from any addiction, just turn that fear into faith, and God will, for Christ sake, save, deliver, and set you free from this obsession to use alcohol and other drugs. Many believe, as long as they join a church, and be put on the membership role or book, that is the answer. The answer is Christ. The Apostle Paul said in II Corinthians 5: 17, "Therefore if any man be in Christ, he is a new creature: old things are passed away; behold, all things are become new."

I would argue, having your name on a church membership role, doesn't save you. Man needs a relationship with his creator (God), and the key in this process is (Jesus Christ). In the book of Romans 10:9,10 Paul said," That if thou shalt confess with thy mouth the Lord Jesus, and shalt believe in thine heart God hath raised him from the dead, thou shalt be saved. For with the heart man believeth unto righteousness; and with the mouth confession is made unto salvation."

In the book of Hebrews 7:25, "Wherefore he is able also to save them to the uttermost that come unto God by him, seeing he ever liveth to make intercession for them." It doesn't matter what kind of life you are living in sin, God is able and will save and deliver you from sin and death, if you only can believe. Jesus said himself, Luke 19:10," For the Son of man is come to seek and to save that which was lost."

Many people are anxious and they are experiencing a great deal of anxiety because of a life of sin. Unless they are born with this disorder. But, to the man or women, who are depressed and full of anxiety, I recommend (Jesus) to you, St. matthew 6:25," Therefore I say unto you, Take no thought for your life, what ye shall eat, or what ye shall drink; nor yet for your body, what ye shall put on. Is not the life more than meat, and the body than raiment?."

Sometimes we continue to suffer because, we never thought about praying and asking god to forgive us of our sins, and to save us. St. matthew 7: 7, Jesus said," Ask, and it shall be given you; seek, and ye shall find; knock, and it shall be opened unto you. Verse 8: (For every one that asketh receiveth; and he that seeketh findeth; and to him that knocketh it shall be opened."

In contrast, The book of James said, "But let him ask in faith, nothing wavering. For he that waverth is like a wave of the sea driven with the wind and tossed." James 1:5. If the individual, even though, he or she ask in faith, however, if they really don't believe in what they are asking will be given, they ask in vain.

Many believer's say, "I just can't help it, I am not perfect." We all know, that there is none perfect, said Jesus Christ. However, James 1:13, says "let no man say when he is tempted, I am tempted of God; for God cannot be tempted with evil, neither tempteth he any man: Vs. 14. "But every man is tempted, when he is drawn away of his own lust, and enticed. Vs. 15. "Then when lust hath conceived, it bringeth forth sin:, when it is finished, bringeth forth death."

This whole salvation process, is all about faith, without faith, "it is impossible to please God." (Heb.11:6, "But without faith it is impossible to please him: for he that cometh to God must believe that he is, and that he is a rewarder of them that diligently seek him." II Cor 5:7, says, "For we walk by faith, not by sight:" The Apostle Paul said in, II Cor 4: 3-5, "But if our gospel be hid, it is hid to them that are lost. In whom the god of this world (satan) hath blinded the minds of them which believe not, lest the light of the glorious gospel of Christ, who is the image of God, should shine unto them. For we preach not ourselves, but Christ Jesus the Lord; and ourselves your servants for Jesus sake."

I feel like preaching right about now, for the sake of those, who may not, or have a problem, believing in the Gospel of Jesus Christ, for it is not about us, (preacher/messenger), but about the Lord and Savior Jesus Christ, he doeth the work. Paul said in Romans 1:15-16," So, as much as in me is, I am ready to preach the gospel to you that are at Rome also. Vs 16, "For I am not ashamed of the gospel of Christ: for it is the power of God unto salvation to everyone that believeth; to the Jew first, and also to the Greek."

Many in Christ, and in the visible (Church), are confused, If you or we, are not in Christ, having our name on the membership role in our local Church, do not mean anything. We must be in Christ, in order to be saved. When the believer accepts Christ as his or her Savior, he or she takes on the Spirit of Christ, and it is his (Jesus Christ) Spirit that saves us, and keeps us saved, until the day of redemption. Ephesians 4:30-32," And grieve not the Holy Spirit of God, whereby ye are sealed unto the day of redemption. Let all bitterness and wrath, and anger, and clamour, and evil speaking, be put away from you, with all malice: And be ye kind one to another, tenderhearted, forgiving one another, even as God for Christ sake hath forgiven you."

## "THE WARFARE OF SPIRIT FILLED BELIEVERS"

Paul talked about this in Ephesians 6:10-17, "Finally, my brethren, be strong in the Lord, and in the power of his might. Put on the whole armour of God, that ye may be able to stand against the wiles of the devil. For we wrestle not against flesh and blood, but against principalities, against powers, against the rulers of the darkness of this world, against spiritual wickedness in high places. Wherefore take unto you the whole armour of God, that ye may be able to withstand in the evil day, and having done all, to stand.

Stand therefore, having your loins girt about with truth, and having on the breastplate of righteousness; And your feet shod with the preparation of the gospel of peace; Above all, taking the shield of faith, wherewith ye shall be able to quench all the fiery darts of the wicked. And take the helmet of salvation, and the sword of the spirit, which is the word of God."

In Ephesians 5: 19-21 Paul said," Speaking to yourselves in psalms and hymns and spiritual songs, singing and making melody in your heart to the Lord. Giving thanks always for all things unto God and the Father in the name of our Lord Jesus Christ; Submitting yourselves one to another in the fear of God. Ephesians 5: 9-14, Paul said, "For the fruit of the Spirit is in all goodness and righteousness and truth; proving what is acceptable unto the Lord. And have no fellowship with the unfruitful works of darkness, but rather reprove them. But in all things that are reproved are made manifest by the light: for whatsoever doth make manifest is light. Wherefore he saith, Awake thou that sleepest, and arise from the dead, and Christ shall give thee light."

It is amazing how, when you know the Lord, and meditate on his word, how he (Christ) just ministers to his people. Those who do not know the Lord, are considered dead spiritually speaking, but the Lord can and will ignite the very fiber of our souls, when we surrender to his will and purpose for our lives. I am reminded of another scripture in which Paul wrote about the new life in Christ Jesus. In Galatians 6: 9, he said, "And let us not be weary in well doing; for in due season, we shall reap, if we faint not."

Sometimes, when we seek the Lord for something in particular, and he doesn't answer as early as we anticipate, we have to be aware, God has his own time table for everything, including us. So whatever this means for someone who may be reading this book. The above scripture was just put in my spirit to write. But just remember, Wait on the Lord, and be of good cheer, for he will answer our request and petitions in due time. He may not come when we want him, but he is right on time.

There are times that, we need to do what Paul said in Hebrews 12: 1-2, "Wherefore seeing we also are compassed about with so great a cloud of witness, let us lay aside every weight, and the sin which doth so easily beset us, and let us run with patience the race that is set before us. Looking unto Jesus the Author and finisher of our faith; who for the joy that was set before him endured the cross, despising the shame, and is set down at the right hand of the throne of God."

Some, who may choose to read this book, have troubled hearts, Jesus had something for you also. St. John 14: 1-2, "Let not your heart be troubled: ye believe in God, believe also in me. In my Father's house are many mansions: if it were not so, I would have told you. I go to prepare a place for you. Vs. 3. And if I go and prepare a place for you, I will come again, and receive you unto myself; that where I am, there ye may be also.

When an individual gives his or her heart to the Lord, it is amazing how, the suffering that we once experienced, will disappear. Although, there may be some suffering we as believer's may go through, suffering as a Christian, We that live Godly in Christ Jesus may suffer, however, this kind of suffering cannot be compared with the suffering of a sinful life. Jesus said, St. John 10:10, "The thief cometh not, but for to steal, and to kill, and to destroy: I am come that they might have life, and that they might have it more abundantly."

Jesus Christ can supply all of your needs. In Philippians 4: 19, Paul told the Church at Philippi, "But my God shall supply all your need according to his riches in glory by Christ Jesus. The word of God said this, and if the word of God said it, that should settle it. For God cannot lie, and will not lie. Paul also said, "I can do all things through Christ which strengtheneth me." (Philippians 4: 13.)

Many might say, "God would never save me, based on my present and former life. Well, I beg the difference with you. This is why Christ came. In St. Luke 19: 10, Jesus said," For the Son of man is come to seek and to save that which was lost. "In St. Luke 2: 17, Jesus said," When Jesus heard it, he saith unto them, They that are whole have no need of the physician, but they that are sick: I came to not to call the righteous, but sinners to repentance."

## "PSYCHOLOGICAL SUFFERING"

many today, in these last and evil times in the Christian arena, many are suffering in their mind. This brings about, diffusion, confusion, and sometimes bizarre behavior. They may ask, "What can God do for me.?" I am glad you asked, II Timothy 1:7, Paul said, "For God hath not given us the spirit of fear; but of power, and of love, and of a sound mind." God doesn't give man, a confused mind. Sin is basically the reason for a mind that is out of balance. Sometimes the sin of the parents, or, sins of the person, however, this kind of population was not originally created by God.

In the book of Genesis, the first chapter, deals with God creating the original creation of the heaven and Earth, Gen1: 1-2. Vs. 3-4 deals with light and darkness. Vs. 5 deals with differentiation of day (light), and night (darkness). The third day, deals with land and sea, vs, 9-10.

The fourth day deals with the Sun, Moon and Stars. Gen 1: 14-19, these all became visible to man. The fifth day, the second creative act-animal life. Vs. 20-23, And God said, "let the Earth bring forth the living creature after his kind, cattle, and creeping thing, and beast of the earth after his kind, and cattle after their kind, and every thing that creepeth upon the earth after his kind: and God saw that it was good.

The sixth day: The creation of man; Gen 1:26, "And God said, let us make man in our image, after our likeness: and let them have dominion over the fish of the sea, and over the fowl of the air, and over the cattle, and over all the earth, and over every creeping thing that creepeth upon the earth." Vs. 27 "So God created man in his own image, in the image of God created he him, male and female created he them."

In Vs. 28: God said, "And God blessed them, and God said unto them, Be fruitful, and multiply, and replenish the earth, and subdue it: and have dominion over the fish of the sea, and over the fowl of the air, and over every living thing that moveth upon the earth. "vs. 31" And God saw every thing that he had made, and behold, it was very good. And the evening and the morning were the sixth day.

In II Tim1: 7, "For God hath not given us the spirit of fear; but of power, and of love, and of a sound mind. "So, if God said that every thing he made was, very good, this means that, Psychological suffering does not come from God, either from a gene, or genectic, from one's own parent, or from a sinful life. God really honored his creation of man, if you read the 8th Psalm Vs. 4-9, "What is man, that thou art mindful of him? And the son of man, that thou visitest him?

For thou hast made him a little lower than the angels, and hast crowned him with glory and honour. Thou madest him to have dominion over the works of thy hands; thou hast put all things under his feet; All sheep and oxen, yea, and the beasts of the field; The fowl of the air, and the fish of the sea, and whatsoever passeth through the paths of the seas. O Lord our Lord, how excellent is thy name in all the earth.

Now, you see why God did not make a psychological misfit of a man. Just think about the verse that says, "For thou hast made him a little lower than the angels, and hast crowned him with glory and honour. So, if man has been crowned with glory and honour, to worship, glorify, and honor his creator, (God) can't and will not, make his creation suffer like this, only sin and satan makes man a psychological misfit.

## "MENTAL SUFFERING"

Many people go through mental suffering, some on a daily basis, and some, periodically, maybe once a week or twice a month. I am reminded what King Solomon said in Proverbs 23: 7, "For as he thinketh in his heart, so is he: Eat and drink, saith he to thee; but his heart is not with thee." The mind of man operates from a belief system. Some of our beliefs are based on what we have been exposed to in our earlier environment.

For example, e.g.; if a person has been exposed to abuse in their home environment, and most of the time, they have to hide behind a chair or sofa to protect themselves, this individual will have a tendency to hide from reality. They will start to use an ego-defense mechanism call denial. By using this defense, they protect the inner self from harm or danger. Although this, for the most part is used unconsciously, it works for the person most of the time.

Just because we operate from a belief system, this doesn't mean that this system is always correct. Take the drug addict, or alcoholic, and think about how this individual continues to do the same thing, but expects a different result. This person is in denial that this kind of behavior will work for him or her for the better. However, if this person will only check out the results of this kind of behavior, they will find that, if nothing changes, nothing changes.

Even though this person or persons, are told you have to change one thing, everything. This person with this kind of thinking will continue the same thinking, and as a consequence, the results are always the same. They will lose their job, family, health, and sometime even their minds, if they continue to drink or drug. Notwithstanding, they sometimes will also get arrested for drunk driving, burglary, armed robbery, etc;.

You might say. "What does it take for a person to learn from their mistakes.?" Well that depends on the mindset of the person involved." If I do not tell anyone what I am going to do, maybe this will work the next time. This person is operating from a (pseudo) belief system. A false belief, that they can still execute the same behavior, but have a different result. It is not going to happen.

There is a self- help program that teaches, made a decision to turn my will and my life over to the care of God, as I understand him. It will not work, unless you do what the step says. Turn both over to the care of God. What you are saying to yourself is, I can't do it, so I believe God can, and I will let him. God can do for man, what man can't do for himself. Many have tried to do it there way, but it never seems to work for them.

The mental suffering from this kind of behavior is real and gives negative rewards. Hospitals, Psy-wards, Jail, prison, and sometimes death. In proverbs 15: 22. "Without counsel purposes are disappointed: but in the multitude of counselors they are established." Proverbs 21:30 says, "There is no wisdom nor understanding nor counsel against the Lord. "God gives wisdom to them that seek it, and those that seek it, most of the time, will share it. But guess what?, Can't make another human being accept it, (the truth).

Proverbs 20: 1, says "Wine is a mocker, strong drink is raging: and whosoever is deceived thereby is not wise." It is amazing how, we might say to ourselves, "I will never ever put myself in this position again, however, because of the addiction process, the addict or alcoholic responds to his or her addiction needs first, and everything after that is secondary. I know this is tight, but it is right. Sometimes man can hear the truth, but until man decides to accept the truth, he or she will continue to go through the same mental, emotional changes and will suffer.

Proverbs 21: 2, "Every way of a man is right in his own eyes: but the Lord pondereth the hearts." The mental anguish behind mental suffering is devastating, in terms of, a person may asked themselves," Why do I keep doing the same thing, and why do I keep thinking, things are going to be different." The only way things will change, is when we decide to listen to learn, and learn to listen, and then take appropriate action. Proverbs 26: 12, "Seest thou a man wise in his own conceit? There is more hope of a fool than of him."

When a person has stinking thinking, they wind up, stinking. Well think about it, My thinking got me in most of my trouble, when I was drinking alcoholically, and using marijuana, or should I say, abusing marijuana. The mental obsession to drink and to use marijuana was unreal for me. There were many mornings I would wake up and say to myself, "I am not going to drink today, and not smoke today, and guess what?, I still dranked and smoked because of my obsession to use a chemical."

There are three phases of suffering from an addiction. There is the Mental, the Physical, and the Spiritual. The recovery process will not necessarily, be in the same order, however, when God deliver a person from this addiction, the process of recovery begins. I had mentioned earlier about the psychological, I just finished about the mental, I will now discuss the physical aspect.

I would like to start with the layout of the Nervous system, the author of this very complexed text, deserves a great deal of credit for his research and knowledge, he so graciously shared with us students of Psychology. First of all, the average person is not cognizant, of what happens to them when they induce a chemical in their blood stream. Now, I will share what has been explored and proven in science in this textbook. At least some of the major concepts, theory and proven results. The author is (John P. J. Pinel), The title of the textbook is, BIOPSYCHOLOGY. Copyright 2003, 5th edition.

## "DIVISIONS OF THE NERVOUS SYSTEM"

The central nervous system (CNS) is the division of the nervous system that is located within the skull and spine. The peripheral nervous system (PNS) is the division that is located outside the skull and spine. The central nervous system is composed of two divisions: the brain and the spinal cord. The brain is the part of the CNS that is located in the skull; the Spinal Cord is the part that is located in the spine.

The Peripheral nervous system is also composed of two divisions: The Somatic nervous system and the autonomic nervous system. The somatic nervous system (SNS) is the part of the PNS THAT INTERACTS WITH THE EXTERNAL ENVIRONMENT. It is composed of Afferent nerves that carry sensory signals from the skin, skeletal muscles, joints, eyes, ears, and so on to the central nervous system, and the Efferent nerves that carry motor signals from the central nervous system to the skeletal muscles.

The Autonomic nervous system (ANS) is the part of the peripheral nervous system that participates in the regulation of the internal environment. It is composed of Afferent nerves that carry sensory signals from internal organs to the (CNS) and efferent nerves that carry motor signals from the (CNS) to internal organs. The autonomic nervous system has two kinds of efferent nerves: sympathetic nerves and parasympathetic nerves

The conventional view of the respective functions of the sympathetic and parasympathetic systems stresses three important principles: (1) That sympathetic nerves stimulate, organize, and mobilize energy resources in threatening situations, whereas parasympathetic nerves act to conserve energy; (2) That each autonomic target organ receives opposing sympathetic and parasympathetic input, and its activity is thus controlled by relative levels of sympathetic and parasympathetic activity; and (3) That sympathetic changes are indicative of psychological arousal, whereas parasympathetic changes are indicative of psychological relaxation.

Although these principles are generally correct, there are significant exceptions to each of them. The brain and spinal cord (the CNS) are the most protected organs in the body. They are encased in bone and covered by three protective membranes, the three (MENINGES), The outer (MENINX) which is the singular of meninges called the DURA MATER. Also protecting the CNS is the cerebrospinal fluid (CSF), which fills the subarachnoid space.

## "THE FIVE MAJOR DIVISIONS OF THE BRAIN"

The five swellings that compose the developing brain at birth are the (Telencephalon), The (Diencephalon), The (Mesencephalon), The (Metencephalon), and the (Myelencephalon). These swellings ultimately develop into the five divisions of the adult brain. An interesting part of the myelencephalon from a psychological perspective is the (Reticular Formation), The reticular formation plays a role in arousal. Also, including sleep, attention, movement, the maintenance of muscle tone, and various cardiac, circulatory, and respiratory reflexes. (Pinel, John P. J.)

The (Metencephalon), has many descending tracts and part of the reticular formation. These structures create a bulge, called the (Pons), on the brain stem' ventral surface. The Pons is one major division of the Metencephalon; the other is the cerebellum called (the little brain). The cerebellum is the large convoluted structure on the brain stem's dorsal surface. It is an important sensorimotor structure; cerebellar damage eliminates the ability to precisely control one's movements and to adapt them to changing conditions.

However, the fact that cerebellar damage also produces a variety of cognitive deficits suggest that the function of the cerebellum is not restricted to sensorimotor control. The mesencephalon, like the metencephalon, has two divisions. The two divisions of the mesencephalon are the (Tectum) and the (Tegmentum). The tectum is the dorsal surface of the midbrain. In mammals, the tectum is composed of two pairs of bumps, the Colliculi (Little Hills).

The posterior pair, called the 9 Inferior Colliculi, have an auditory function; the anterior pair, called the (Superior Colliculi), have a visual function. In lower vertebrates, the function of the tectum is entirely visual; thus, the tectum is referred to as the optic tectum. The (Diencepephalon) is composed of two structures: the (Thalamus) and the (Hypothalamus). The thalamus is the large, two-lobed structure that constitutes the top of the brain stem.

The (Hypothalmus) is located just below the anterior thalamus. It plays an important role in the regulation of several motivated behaviors. It exerts its effects in part by regulating the release of hormones from the (Pituitary Gland), which dangles from it on the ventral surface of the brain. In addition to the pituitary gland, two other structures appear on the inferior surface of the hypothalamus: The optic chiasm and the mammillary bodies.

The optic chiasm is the point at which the optic nerves from each eye come together. The X shape is created because some of the axons of the optic nerve decussate (cross over to the other side of the brain) via the optic chiasm. The (Telencephalon) is the largest division of the human brain, and it mediates its most complex functions. It initiates voluntary movement, interprets sensory in-put, and mediates complex cognitive processes such as (learning, speaking, and problem solving). (Pinel, John P.J.)

# "BASIC PRINCIPLES OF DRUG ACTION"

I wanted to set up this next section, to let those that choose to continue to suffer from their addiction processes, know what they are doing to their brain, in terms of, the damage from alcohol abuse and other mind altering chemicals. I felt compelled to inform the readers of this book, the danger of such behavior. I will now begin to inform you of what lies ahead of the abuser.

Drug addiction is a serious problem in most parts of the world. For example, in the United States alone, over 60 million people are addicted to nicotine, alcohol, or both; 5.5 million are addicted to illegal drugs; and many millions more are addicted to prescription drugs. Pause for a moment and think about the sheer magnitude of the grief represented by such figures, hundreds of millions of sick and suffering people world wide.

Drugs are usually administered in one of four ways: by oral ingestion, by injection, by inhalation, or by absorption through the mucous membranes of the nose, mouth, or rectum. The route of administration influences the rate at which and the degree to which the drug reaches its sites of action. (INGESTION). The oral route is the preferred route of administration for many drugs. Once they are swallowed, drugs dissolve in the fluids of the stomach and are carried to the intestine, where they are absorbed into the bloodstream.

Its main disadvantage is its unpredictability: absorption from the digestive tract into the bloodstream can be greatly influenced by such difficult-to-gauge factors as the amount and type of food in the stomach. (INJECTION) Drug injection is common in medical practice because the effects of injected drugs are strong, fast, and predictable. Drug injections are typically made subcutaneously (SC), into the fatty tissue just beneath the skin; intramuscularly (IM), into the large muscles; or intravenously (IV), directly into veins at points where they run just beneath the skin.

Many addicts prefer the intravenous route because the bloodstream delivers the drug directly to the brain. However, the speed and directness of the intravenous route are mixed blessings; after an intravenous injection, there is little or no opportunity to counteract the effects of an overdose, an impurity, or an allergic reaction. Futhermore, many addicts develop scar tissue, infections, and collapsed veins at the few sites on their bodies where there are large accessible veins.

Absorption through (Mucous Membranes): Some drugs can be administered through the mucous membranes of the nose, mouth, and rectum. Cocaine, for example, is commonly self-administered through the nasal membranes (snorted)-but not without damaging them.

## (DRUG PENETRATION OF THE CENTRAL NERVOUS SYSTEM)

It is very important to know what happens to our central nervous system, once a drug has been induced. Once a drug enters the bloodstream, it is carried in the blood to the blood vessels of the central nervous system. Fortunately, a protective filter, the blood-brain barrier, makes it difficult for many potentially dangerous bloodborne chemicals to pass from the blood vessels of the (CNS) into its neurons.

## "MECHANISMS OF DRUG ACTION"

I would like to anchor here for a minute, I want to elaborate on what happens to the brain, after being induced by a drug. Most addicts, either don't know, or rather could care less, as long as they get their fix. The brain is divided into two parts, the left side of the brain is, (intellect), the right side of the brain is (pleasure principle side). When an addict or alcoholic who abuse alcohol, induces a chemical, it settles on the right side of the brain. The receptors on this side of the brain say, "Give me more" "Give me more".

The unfortunate part of this whole scenario is, the addict or alcoholic, will not worry about nothing, all is well. (right) I don't think so, how can all be well, when the person inducing these chemicals, have no desire to deal with reality. There is a certain euphoria state through this whole process, once that state has been established, the addict or alcoholic is off to the races for more drugs or chemicals, that makes them feel the way they want to feel. This denotes, no worries, no care feelings, no responsibility for your actions or behavior, it is impossible to be responsible for your actions while under the influence of a chemical. The person's vision is distorted, the judgement of this person is impaired, and the person is just out there somewhere in space.

The tolerance of that person is at a very high rate, however, after awhile, the tolerance level will change. The level that one could handle in the past, becomes a level, that the person inducing the chemical began to experience a different reaction, because the tolerance level has changed. Notice what happens, in my next paragraph on this most interesting subject and demise.

## "MECHANISMS OF DRUG ACTION" "DRUG TOLERANCE"

drug tolerance is a state of decreased sensitivity to a drug that develops as a result of exposure to it. Drug tolerance can be demonstrated in two ways: by showing that a given dose of the drug has less effect than it had before drug exposure or by showing that it takes more of the drug to produce the same effect. In essence, what this means is that drug tolerance is a shift in the dose-response curve.

Failure to understand this second point can have tragic consequences for people who think that because they have become tolerant to some effects of a drug (e.g., to the nauseating effects of alcohol or tobacco), they are tolerant to all of them. In fact, tolerance may develop to some effects of a drug while sensitivity to other effects increases-increases in sensitivity to drugs are called sensitization. The third important point about the specificity of drug tolerance is that it is not a unitary phenomenon; that is, there is no single mechanism that underlies all examples of it. When a drug is administered at active doses, many kinds of adaptive changes can occur to reduce its effects.

Two categories of changes underlie drug tolerance: metabolic and functional. Drug tolerance that results from changes that reduce the amount of drug getting to its sites of action is called (Metabolic Tolerance). Drug tolerance that results from changes that reduce the reactivity of the sites of action to the drug is called (Functional Tolerance). (Pinel, John, p.J., 2003)

Tolerance to psychoactive drugs is largely functional. Functional tolerance to psychoactive drugs can result from several different types of neural changes. For example, exposure to a psychoactive drug can reduce the number of receptors for it, decrease the efficiency with which it binds to existing receptors, or diminish the impact of receptor binding on the activity of the cell.

# "DRUG WITHDRAWAL EFFECTS AND PHYSICAL DEPENDENCE"

Individuals who suffer withdrawal reactions when they stop taking taking a drug are said to be physically dependent on that drug. The fact that withdrawal effects are frequently opposite to the initial effects of the drug suggests that withdrawal effects may be produced by the same neural changes that produce drug tolerance. According to this theory, exposure to a drug produces compensatory changes in the nervous system that offset the drug's effects and produce tolerance.

# "ADDICTION: WHAT IS IT?"

Addicts are habitual drug users, but not all habitual drug users are addicts. Addicts are those habitual drug users who continue to use a drug despite its adverse effects on their health and social life and despite their repeated efforts to stop using it. The greatest confusion about the nature of addiction concerns its relation to physical dependence. Many people equate the two.

If it were, addicts could be easily cured by hospitalizing them for a few days, until their withdrawal symptoms subsided. However, most addicts renew their drug taking even after months of enforced abstinence. This is an important issue, and it will be revisited later in the chapter. When physical dependence was believed to be the major cause of addiction, the term psychological dependence was coined to refer to exceptions to this general rule.

# "FIVE COMMONLY ABUSED DRUGS"

TOBACCO: When a cigarette is smoked, nicotine-the major psychoactive ingredient of tobacco-and some 4,000 other chemicals, collectively referred to as tar, are absorbed through the lungs. Approximately 76 million Americans have consumed nicotine in the last month. There is no question that heavy smokers are drug addicts in every sense of the word (Jones, 1987). The compulsive drug craving, which is the major defining feature of addiction, is readily apparent in any habitual smoker who has run out of cigarettes or who is forced by circumstance to refrain from smoking for several hours.

About 70% of all people who experiment with smoking become addicted-this figure compares unfavorably with 10% for alcohol and 30% for heroin. Twin studies (Lerman et al., 1999; true et al., 1999) indicate that nicotine addiction has a major genetic component. The heritability estimate is about 65%. Moreover, only about 20% of all attempts to stop smoking are successful for 2 years or more. (Schelling, 1992).

The adverse effects of tobacco smoke are unfortunately not restricted to those who smoke. There is now strong evidence that individuals who live or work with smokers are more likely to develop heart disease and cancer: Smoking during pregnancy increases the likelihood of miscarriage, stillbirth, and early death of the child. The levels of nicotine in the blood of breastfed infants are often as great as those in the blood of their smoking mothers.

## "ALCOHOL"

Approximately 104 million Americans have consumed alcohol in the last month, 13 million of these are heavy users, and over 100,000 die each year from alcohol-related diseases and accidents. Alcohol is involved in roughly 3% of all deaths in the United States, including deaths from birth defects, ill health, accidents, and violence. Because alcohol molecules are small and soluble in both fat and water, they invade all parts of the body. Alcohol is classified as a depressant because at moderate-to-high doses it depresses neural firing.

"The Killer Drug," and "Marijuana Madness." The population was told that marijuana turns normal people into violent, drug-crazed criminals who rapidly become addicted to heroin. The result of the misrepresentation of the effects of marijuana by the U.S. news media was the enactment of many laws against the drug. In many states, marijuana was legally classified a narcotic (a legal term generally used to refer to opiates), and punishment for its use was dealt out accordingly.

However, the structure of the active constituents of marijuana and their physiological and behavioral effects bear no resemblance to those of the other narcotics; thus, legally classifying marijuana as a narcotic was akin to passing a law that red is green. The popularization of marijuana smoking among the middle and upper class in the 1960s stimulated a massive program of research; yet there is still considerable confusion about marijuana among the general population. One of the difficulties in characterizing the effects of marijuana is that they are subtle, difficult to measure, and greatly influenced by the social situation:

However, even after high doses, an unexpected knock at the door can often bring about the return of a reasonable semblance of normal behavior. In the light of the documented effects of marijuana, the earlier claims that marijuana would trigger a wave of violent crimes in the youth of America seem absurd. It is difficult to imagine how anybody could believe that the red-eyed, gluttonous, sleepy, giggling products of common social doses of marijuana would be likely to commit violent criminal acts. In fact, marijuana actually curbs aggressive behavior (Tinklenberg, 1974).

What are the hazards of long-term marijuana use? The main problems appear to be respiratory, (Zimmer & Morgan, 1997). The minority of marijuana smokers who continually smoke the drug tend to have deficits in respiratory function (e. g., Tilles et al., 1986), and they are more likely to develop a chronic cough, bronchitis, and asthma (Abramson, 1974).

## "COCAINE AND OTHER STIMULANTS"

Stimulants are drugs whose primary effect is to produce general increases in neural and behavioral activity. Although stimulants all have a similar profile of effects, they differ greatly in their potency. Coca-Cola is a mild commercial stimulant preparation consumed by many people around the world. Today, its stimulant action is attributable to caffeine, but when it was first introduced, "the pause that refreshes" packed a real wallop in the form of small amounts of cocaine. Cocaine and its derivatives are the most commonly abused stimulants, and thus they are the focus of this discussion.

Cocaine hydrochloride may be converted to its base form by boiling it in a solution of baking soda until the water has evaporated. The impure residue of this process is crack, which is a potent, cheap, smokable form of cocaine. Crack has rapidly become the preferred form of the drug for many cocaine users. However, because crack is impure, variable, and consumed by smoking, it is difficult to study and most research on cocaine derivatives has thus focused on pure cocaine hydrochloride. Approximately 1.5 million Americans used cocaine or crack in the last month.

Like alcohol, cocaine hydrochloride is frequently consumed in binges (Gawin, 1991). Cocaine addicts tend to go on so-called cocaine sprees, binges in which extremely high levels of intake are maintained for periods of a day or two. During a cocaine spree, users become increasingly tolerant to the euphoria-producing effects of cocaine. Accordingly, larger and larger doses are often administered. The spree usually ends when the cocaine is gone or when it begins to have serious toxic effects.

Extremely high blood levels of cocaine are reached during cocaine sprees The results commonly include sleeplessness, tremors, nausea, and psychotic behavior. The syndrome of psychotic behavior observed during cocaine sprees is called cocaine psychosis. It is similar to, and has often been mistakenly diagnosed as, Paranoid Schizophrenia. During cocaine sprees, there is a risk of loss of consciousness and death from seizures (Earnest, 1993), respiratory arrest, or stroke (Kokkinos & Levine, 1993).

Although cocaine is extremely addictive, the withdrawal effects triggered by abrupt termination of a cocaine spree are mild (Miller, Summers, & Gold, 1993). Common cocaine withdrawal symptoms include a negative mood swing and insomnia. Cocaine facilitates catecholaminergic transmission. It does this by blocking the reuptake of catecholamines (dopamine, norepinephrine, and epinephrine) into pre-synaptic neurons. Its effects on dopaminergic transmission seem to play the major role in mediating its euphoria-inducing effects.

Cocaine and its derivatives are not the only commonly abused stimulants. AMPHETAMINE (speed) and its relatives also present major health problems.

This next section is very important, in terms of, how drugs influence synaptic transmission. Although the synthesis, release, and action of neurotransmitters vary somewhat from neurotransmitter to neurotransmitter (Walmsley, Alvarez, & Fyffe, 1998). Psychoactive drugs: Cocaine is a potent catecholamine agonist that is highly addictive. It increases the activity of both dopamine and norepinephrine by blocking their reuptake from the synapse into the presynaptic button.

Accordingly, when there are high levels of cocaine in the brain, molecules of dopamine and norepinephrine, once released into the synapse, continue to activate postsytivation has been blocked. This produces a variety of psychological effects, including euphoria, loss of appetite, and insomnia. It is also responsible for the addictive potential of cocaine. Now thinking about and wondering in amazement how God made man in his own image. Our brain already have natural chemicals imputed there from birth. Part of the brains function is to, receive messages, as well as, transmit messages.

Any interruption of this natural process, causes confusion in the brain's receptor sites, and thus, these synaptic transmissions are delayed or are eliminated from its normal processes. When an individual induces a drug into his or her blood stream, which ordinarily doesn't belong there, for the most part, the drug usually rest on the right side of the brain, which is the pleasure principle receptor. When this happens, the receptors begin to say to the drug, give me more, give me more, as a result of this process, a state of euphoria is experienced. (which is a well being state of elation, or un-natural high).

I would like to inject another concept, which I believe most people who uses drugs are not cognizant of, which is, by doing things right, and being responsible for exhibiting good patterns of behavior, man is automatically rewarded by a feeling of accomplishment, in turn, which puts him or her, in a natural state of a high or elation. Man do not need a drug to go on a trip to no where, not knowing where he will land, if he or she will land at all in an appropriate place. The chemicals, which God created man with, are plenty enough to experience a good feeling about one's self.

One thing is for sure, you will know where you went, what happened, and how you got home. Under the influence of drugs and abuse of alcohol or amphetamines, the individual's vision is obscure (hidden by darkness, not able to clearly see, not readily understood, or indistinct). Why would anyone want to experience this constant confused state, every time they get high.? I guess this population just like to suffer, or should I say, choose to suffer.

God made man with all of the necessary equipment to function and operate in the world he made first, and then man. Maybe, it was a good thing that God made his world first, and then man to live in it (world). I just want the reader to peruse this concept. God gave man a brain, man is a free moral agent, he has a choice to do what he or she chooses to do, man has a brain to think from, eyes to see, mouth with teethe to eat and talk from, fingers to feel, legs and feet to walk, and a decision making process, to chose his or her behavior from. The lower animal is not equipped with this kind of mechanism.

Now why, would man take something that is so wonderfully made by God his (Creator), and contaminate it with his or her never satisfied mindset.? Take advantage of what the lower animal doesn't have, never intended for him to have in the first place, and appreciate what you are. Paul said, in Romans 12: 1, "I beseech you therefore, brethren, by the mercies of God, that ye present your bodies a living sacrifice, holy, acceptable unto God, which is your reasonable service." I feel like preaching right about now.

Why, contaminate something so wonderfully made like yourself, with foreign substances, such as alcohol, marijuana, cocaine, amphetamines, heroin, etc,. Job 5: 17, "Behold, happy is the man whom God correcteth: therefore despise not thou the chastening of the almighty." I would not have the ability to write what I am writing now, if I had not accept the chastening of the Lord God. For sure, I would have left this beautiful life, many years ago, and would not be able to help somebody else, who might be receptive to the truth. Speaking of truth, Jesus said in St. John 14:6," Jesus saith unto him, I am the way, the truth and the life: no man cometh unto the Father, but by me."

To put it succinctly, (to the point without wasted words) Romans 6: 23 says," For the wages of sin is death; but the gift of God is eternal life through Jesus Christ our Lord." Why pay for death, when salvation is free, through Jesus Christ our Lord. Romans 6: 16, Paul said, "Know ye not, that to whom ye yield yourselves servants to obey, his servants ye are to whom ye obey; whether of sin unto death, or of obedience unto righteousness.?"

I just wanted to get that little message across to the reader of these pages, trust me, this is real good reading, because the author has experienced, which is empirical knowledge, what he is writing, to a state of victory in Jesus, I know from whence I speak, like Paul said in Romans 8:38," For I am persuaded, that neither death, nor life, nor angels, nor principalities, nor powers, nor things present, nor things to come. Vs. 39, nor height, nor depth, nor any other creature, shall be able to separate us from the love of God, which is in Christ Jesus our Lord." Think about this, all of this Christian walk in life is free, all you have to do is just believe, and if you can believe the gospel of Jesus Christ, and that he was crucified, died, and resurrected on the third day, according to the scriptures, thou shalt be saved.

Romans 10:9-10, "That if thou shalt confess with thy mouth the Lord Jesus, and shalt believe in thine heart that God hath raised him from the dead, thou shalt be saved. For with the heart man believeth unto righteousness; and with the mouth confession is made unto salvation." Romans 10: 17," So then faith cometh by hearing, and hearing by the word of God." So then, if you can believe it, you can receive it. It is all according to your faith. Why not just believe, it is free, it doesn't cost you nothing but your faith. But, think about what you gain, eternal life, and a life of goodness and kindness, even before you go to meet your savior (Jesus Christ).

## "BIOPSYCHOLOGICAL THERORIES OF ADDICTION"

Early drug addiction treatment programs were based on the physical-dependence theory of addiction. They attempted to break the vicious circle of drug taking by gradually withdrawing drugs from addicts in a hospital environment. Unfortunately, once discharged, almost all detoxified addicts return to their former drug-taking habits-detoxed addicts are addicts who have no drugs in their bodies and who are no longer experiencing withdrawal symptoms.

However, whether detoxification is by choice or necessity, it does not stop addicts from renewing their drug-taking habits (Leshner, 1997). A more recent physical-dependence theory of drug addiction attempts to account for the fact that addicts frequently relapse after lengthy drug-free periods by pointing to the fact that withdrawal symptoms can be conditioned. According to this theory, when addicts who have remained drug-free for a considerable period of time return to a situation in which they have previously experienced the drug, conditioned withdrawal effects opposite to the effects of the drug (conditioned compensatory responses) are elicited. These effects are presumed to result in a powerful craving for the drug to counteract them.

The theory that relapse is motivated primarily by an attempt to counteract conditioned withdrawal effects encounters two major problems. One is that many of the effects elicited by environments that have previously been associated with drug administration are similar to those of the drug rather than being antagonistic to them. The second is that experimental animals and addicts often display a preference for drug-predictive cues, even when no drug is forthcoming (e.g., Bozarth & Wise, 1981; Mucha et al., 1982; White, Sklar, & Amit, 1977). (Pinel, John, P.J., 2003).

For example, some detoxified heroin addicts called needle freaks derive pleasure from sticking an empty needle into themselves. It therefore seems unlikely that conditioned withdrawal effects are the major motivating factors in drug relapse. Rats, humans, and many other species will administer brief bursts of electrical stimulation to specific sites in their own brains. This phenomenon is known as intracranial self-stimulation (ICSS), and the brain sites capable of mediating the phenomenon are often called pleasure centers.

There are three natural rewards circuits. First, brain stimulation through electrodes that mediate self-stimulation often elicits a natural motivated behavior such as eating, drinking, maternal behavior, or copulation in the presence of the appropriate goal object. Second, producing increases in natural motivation (for example, by food or water deprivation, by hormone injections, or by the presence of prey objects) often increases self-stimulation rates (e.g., Caggiula, 1970). And third, it became clear that differences between the situations in which the rewarding effects of brain stimulation and those of natural rewards were usually studied contribute to the impression that these effects are qualitavely different.

## "TWO KEY METHODS FOR MEASURING DRUG-PRODUCED REINFORCEMENT"

In the conditioned place-preference paradigm, rats repeatedly receive a drug in one compartment (the drug compartment) of a two-compartment box. Then, during the test phase, the rat is place in the box drug-free, and the proportion of time it spends in the drug compartment, as opposed to the equal-sized but distinctive control compartment, is measured. Rats usually prefer the drug compartment over the control compartment when the drug compartment has been associated with the effects of drugs to which humans become addicted. The main advantage of the conditioned place-preference paradigm is that the subjects are tested drug-free, which means that the measure of the incentive value of a drug is not confounded by other effects the drug might have on behavior (Carr, Fibiger, & Phillips, 1989; Van der Kooy, 1987).

## "EVIDENCE OF THE INVOLVEMENT OF DOPAMINE IN DRUG ADDICTION"

This section is very important, in terms of, informing the reader of our natural chemicals, how they play a major role in our addiction process. To begin: Strong evidence that dopamine is involved in the drug-induced pleasure experienced by human addicts comes from the study by Volkow and colleagues (1997). They administered various doses of radioactively labeled cocaine to addicts and asked the addicts to rate the resulting "high". They also used positron emission tomography (PET) to measure the degree to which the labeled cocaine bound to dopamine transporters.

Once evidence had accumulated linking dopamine to natural reinforcers and drug –induced rewards, investigators began to explore particular sites in the mesocorticolimbic dopamine pathway. Their findings soon focused attention on the nucleus accubens. Events occurring in the nucleus accumbens and dopaminergic input to it from the ventral tegmental area most clearly related to the experience of reward and pleasure. The following are four of the findings from research on laboratory animals that focused attention on the nucleus accumbens (Ikemoto & Panksepp, 1999; Spanagel & Weiss, 1999):

1. Laboratory animals self-administered microinjections of addictive drugs (e.g., cocaine, amphetamine, and morphine) directly into the nucleus accumbens.
2. Microinjections of addictive drugs into the nucleus accumbens produced a conditioned place preference for the compartment in which they were administered (e.g., White & Hiroi, 1993).
3. Lesions to either the nucleus accumbens or the ventral tegmental area blocked the self-administration of drugs into general circulation or the development of drug-associated conditioned place preferences (e.g., Kelsey, Carlezon, & Falls, 1989: Roberts & Koob, 1982; Roberts et al., 1980)

Nucleus Accumbens, as a result of the earlier research done on the subject of addiction, has been verified as the pleasure and reward center in the brain for the addict. That dopaminergic activity of the nucleus accumbens mediated the reinforcing effects of all addictive drugs and natural reinforcers. Most influential in the thinking of researchers about function of the nucleus accumbens have been reports that extracellular dopamine levels in this brain area increase inresponse to stimuli that indicate that a reward will soon be delivered.

The discovery that its extracellular dopamine levels surge in response to stimuli that predict reward suggests that the role of the nucleus accumbens is not to mediate the experience of pleasure but rather to predict pleasure. It is important not to lose sight of the fact that brain mechanisms was not created by God to support addiction; they were created to serve natural adaptive functions and have somehow been co-opted by addictive drugs.

## "BRAIN MECHANISMS OF HUMAN EMOTION"

Most recent studies of the brain mechanisms of emotion in humans are of two types: neuropsychological studies of emotional changes in brain-damaged patients (Kolb & Taylor, 2000) and functional brain-imaging studies of healthy subjects (Dolen & Morris, 2000; Whalen, 1998). The strength of this contemporary research is that it generally confirms and extends the research conducted on nonhumans species. Specifically, recent studies of the brain mechanisms of emotion have repeatedly confirmed the involvement of the Amygdala and the Prefontal Cortex-although they have not been so kind to the Limbic Theory (LeDoux, 2000b; Calder, Lawrence, & Young, 2001).

The results of a PET study of the perception of fear from prosody make a similar point (Morris, Scott, & Dolan, 1999) The right amygdala and right prefrontal cortex responded more to fearful speech than did their left-hemisphere counterparts, but the right temporal lobe responded less than the left temporal lobe. Consequently, when you think of someone under the influence of a drug induced chemical, (e.g., cocaine, alcohol, or amphetamine) and they decide to attack someone in order to get money to do more drugs, what is to say that, they may not even be warn by an emotion because, that part of the brain to warn them, have been polluted with drugs.

For instance, take a person under the influence of a drug to the degree, that they really are not in reality. It is possible, this person could be diagnosed to be (Schizophrenic), please do not misunderstand this concept. There are people who really have been diagnosed schizophrenic, who really are sick. Why I said this is to help alcoholic's and maybe other addicts, realize, if you give up the drug, you may discover, that you really are not sick at all. Now, on the other hand, if you continue the same behavior after not using any drugs, you do the math.

The term schizophrenia means the splitting of psychic functions. The term was coined in the early 1900s to describe what was assumed at that time to be the primary symptom of the disorder: the breakdown of integration among emotion, thought, and action. Schizophrenia is the disease that is most commonly associated with the concept of madness. It attacks about 1% of individuals of all races and cultural groups, typically beginning in adolescence or early adulthood.

Inappropriate affect. Failure to react with an appropriate level of emotionality to positive or negative events (Keltner, Kring, & Bonanno, 1999; Kring, 1999). Hallucinations. Imaginary voices telling the person what to do or commenting negatively on the person's behavior. Incoherent thought. Illogical thinking, peculiar associations among ideas, or belief in supernatural forces. Odd behavior. Long periods with no movement (catatonia), a lack of personal hygiene, talking in rhymes, avoiding social interaction, echolia.

From research, it is suggested that, a disruption of dopamineric transmission might produce Parkinson's disease and, because of the relation between Parkinson's disease and the antischizophrenic effects of chlorpromazine and reserpine, also suggested that antischizophrenic drug effects might be produced in the same way. Thus was born the dopamine theory of schizophrenia-the theory that schizophrenia is caused by too much dopamine and, conversely, that antischizophrenic drugs exert their effects by decreasing dopamine levels.

Some of the most brilliant people in the world, have been diagnosed with schizophrenia. You might ask me then. How do these people function in their brilliant talent, etc;?. The answer is very simple, by taking their prescribed medication. There is hope for many people, who have been diagnosed with different disorders. The main ingredient for a person like this, to follow their medication regiment. Most patient's with disorders, besides taking their meds, usually go into psychotherapy as well. The combination of both, meds, and therapy, usually works for the best.

# "RECOVERY OF FUNCTION AFTER BRAIN DAMAGE"

Understanding the mechanisms that underlie the recovery of function after nervous system damage is a high priority for neuroscientists. If these mechanisms were understood, steps could be taken to promote recovery, however, recovery of function after nervous system damage is a poorly understood phenomenon. Little is known about recovery of function after nervous system damage for two reasons.

The first is that it is difficult to conduct controlled experiments on populations of brain-damage patients. The second is that nervous system damage may result in a variety of compensatory changes that can easily be confused with true recovery of function. For example, any improvement in the week or two after damage could reflect a decline in cerebral edema (brain swelling) rather than a recovery from the neural damage itself, and any gradual improvement in the months after damage could reflect the learning of new cognitive and behavioral strategies (i.e., substitution of functions) rather than the return of lost functions, (Wilson, 1998). (pinel, John P.J., 2003).

The main thing that I would say to a person, or persons, who were not born, genectically speaking with a disorder, (e.g., Alcoholic, Substance Abuser, etc; remember what the suffering is like, and that it is not going to change for the better, as long as this person continues to abuse drugs. We owe it God our (Creator), and ourselves, to want to be the best person we can be. In terms of, considering our circumstances of course.

# "SUMMARY"

Why people choose to suffer, is a question I wanted to find an answer to, every since I decided to, turn my will and my life over to the care of God, as I understood him. I give this credit to my parents, in terms of, how they introduced God to my sister and I at an early age. Also, the concept of believing in ourselves. It is more profitable for any parent to encourage their children, as oppose to discouraging them. My life was saved many times over I believe, because of my spiritual foundation given to me by my parents, (Rev. Moses Lyons, Jr., and, Nora Hargove Lyons.

Paul said, in Philippians 2: 1-11, "If there be therefore any consolation in Christ, if any comfort of love, if any fellowship of the spirit, if any bowels and mercies. Fulfil ye my joy, that ye be likeminded, having the same love, being of one accord, of one mind. Let nothing be done through strife or vainglory, but in lowliness of mind let each esteem other better than themselves. Look not every man on his own things, but every man also on the things of others.

Let this mind be in you, which was also in Christ Jesus: Who, being in the form of God, thought it not robbery to be equal with God: But made himself of no reputation, and took upon him the form of a servant, and was made in the likeness of men: And being found in fashion as a man, he humbled himself, and became obedient unto death, even the death of the cross. Wherefore God also hath highly exalted him, and given him a name which is above every name:

That at the name of Jesus every knee should bow, of things in heaven, and things in earth, and things under the earth; And that every tongue should confess that Jesus Christ is Lord, to the glory of God the Father: Wherefore, my beloved, as ye have always obeyed, not as in my presence only, but now much more in my absence, work out your own salvation with fear and trembling. Wow, what a servant of the Lord, Paul was. He wanted always to give credit to his ministry, to the honor and glory to the Lord.

This is the only way God can use us, by staying humble at the feet of the cross, and praying for his will to be done in our lives. What are you saying preacher, what I am saying is very simple, "give the credit to the Lord and savior Jesus Christ at all times, and the Lord will raise you up in due time, and will use you for his glory and honor. The problem today is, it seems as God begin to bless us and our Ministries, man gets proud and lifted up, and began to think he is doing this thing. But for the Grace of God, none of us would even be here, in terms of the former life we once led.

God always has, resisted the proud, but giveth grace to the humble. James 4:6, "But he giveth more grace. Wherefore he saith, God resisteth the proud, but giveth grace unto the humble. Vs. 7-8, Submit yourselves therefore to God. Resist the devil, and he will flee from you. Draw nigh to God, and he will draw nigh to you. Cleanse your hands, ye sinners; and purify your hearts, ye double minded.

Sin, is the cause of many illnesses and or sickness. God had and has a remedy for sin, his Son (Jesus Christ). In Romans 3 22-26," Even the righteousness of God which is by faith of Jesus Christ unto all and upon all them that believe: for there is no difference: For all have sinned, and come short of the Glory of God; Being justified freely by his grace through the redemption that is in Christ Jesus: Whom God hath set forth to be a propitiation through faith in his blood, to declare his righteousness for the remission of sins that are past, through the forbearance of God; To declare, I say, at this time his righteousness: that he might be just, and the justifier of him which believeth in Jesus.

In terms of redemption, think about the time, most of us, if we are honest, would go to the pawn shop, and pawn things so we could get money for our addiction purposes. God has a remedy for that, and the name is Jesus Christ. In order to redeem, or get back, what we pawned, you need a ticket, but more importantly, you need the money to redeem back what you pawned. Jesus is man's (Redemption), Jesus is man's propitiation, (sacrifice). The blood of Jesus is what redeems man back to God, his (creator).

In other words, the believing sinner is justified because Christ, having borne his sins on the cross, has been "made unto him righteousness "I Cor 1: 30," But of him are ye in Christ Jesus, who of God is made unto us wisdom, and righteousness, and sanctification, and redemption: God, through his Son (Jesus Christ), did for us who believe, what we could not do for ourselves. Jesus did our dying for us speak that we do know, and testify that we have seen; and ye receive not our witness. If I have told you earthly things, and ye believe not, how shall ye believe, if I tell you of heavenly things? And no man hath ascended up to heaven, but he that came down from heaven, even the Son of man which is in heaven.

And as Moses lifted up the serpent in the wilderness, even so must the Son of man be lifted up: That whosoever believeth in him should not perish, but have eternal life. For God so loved the world, that he gave his only begotten Son, that whosoever believeth in him should not perish, but have everlasting life. (King James Bible).

Some reader's of this book may say, "Why should I think by giving my heart to the Lord Jesus Christ, is going to make a difference in my life.?". Well, I would respond by saying." What do you have to loose. You have everything to gain, at least a much more healthier life, and a life of substance, a life with a positive perspective for once." One might say, "Why, should I believe in something, that I have not seen.?" That is a legimate question, and I submit to you the answer from the scriptures. St. Mark 9: 23, Jesus said, "Jesus said unto him, If thou canst believe, all things are possible to him that believeth."

Jesus prayed to his Father (God), that the father would in the St. John, the 17ᵗʰ chapter, 5-17," And now, O Father, glorify thou me with thine own self with the glory which I had with thee before the world was. I have manifested thy name unto the men which thou gavest me out of the world: thine they were, and thou gavest them to me; and they have kept thy word. Now they have known that all things whatsoever thou hast given me are of thee. (St. James Holy Bible).

For I have given unto them the words which thou gavest me; and they have received them, and have known surely that I came out from thee, and they have believed that thou didst send me. I pray for them: I pray not for the world, but for them which thou hast given me, for they are thine. And all mine are thine, and thine are mine; and I am glorified in them. And now I am no more in the world, but these are in the world, and I come to thee. Holy Father, keep through thine own name those whom thou hast given me, that they may be one, as we are.

While I was with them in the world, I kept them in thy name: those that thou gavest me I have kept, and none of them is lost, but the son of perdition; that the scripture might be fulfilled. And now come I to thee; and these things I speak in the world, that they might have my joy fulfilled in themselves. I have given them thy word; and the world hath hated them, because they are not of the world, even as I am not of the world. I pray not that thou shouldest take them out of the world, but that thou shouldest keep them from the evil. They are not of the world, even as I am not of the world. Sanctify them through thy truth: thy word is truth. (St. James Holy Bible).

Those that may be suffering, and have been for a long time, I give you one more section of scriptures, which should give you a measure of hope, as long as you believe. St. John 16:22-27, Jesus said, "And ye now therefore have sorrow: but I will see you again, and your heart shall rejoice, and your joy no man taketh from you. And in that day ye shall ask me nothing. Verily, verily, I say unto you, Whatsoever ye shall ask the Father in my name, he will give it you. Hitherto have ye asked nothing in my name: ask, and ye shall receive, that your joy may be full.

These things have I spoken unto you in proverbs: but the time cometh, when I shall no more speak unto you in proverbs, but I shall shew you plainly of the Father. At that day ye shall ask in my name: and I say not unto you, that I will pray the Father for you: For the Father himself loveth you, because ye have loved me, and have believed that I came out from God. (St. James Holy Bible).

Apparently, it is time to make a choice, to continue to live beneath your means, or, be willing to accept a remedy that has proven itself for many who accepted Jesus Christ, as there personal Savior. In the book of Joshua 24:15, Joshua said, "And if it seem evil unto you to serve the Lord, choose you this day whom ye will serve. Whether the Gods which your fathers served that were on the other side of the flood, or the gods of the Amorites, in whose land ye dwell: but as for me and my house, we will serve the Lord."

Sometimes, doing what is best for us seems hard and impossible. To some degree you are right, who believe this negative philosophy. The best medicine for us at times, taste the worse, but it gets the job done in the end. David said, In Psalm 34:8, "O taste and see that the Lord is good: blessed is the man that trusteth in him." To those that are still willing to suffer, and continue to exist only, as oppose to having a meaningful life, I pray that if by chance you are reading this book, or hear about it from a friend. Try Jesus, I did and You know what?. Jesus is the most powerful substance that any man can induce, when you induce Jesus, he imputes a spirit of wisdom, knowledge, and understanding that no other human being can possibly give the believer. I tried him, and only because of his blood which he shedded on the cross at Calvary, I am saved delivered and set free today of my addiction to alcohol and other substances. To God, be the glory, today, tomorrow, and forever, AMEN.

Printed in the United States
By Bookmasters